THE

TRUTH

ABOUT

Vitamin E

The Secret to Thriving with Annatto Tocotrienols

BARRIE TAN, PH.D.

Acknowledgments

First, I want to thank my incredibly supportive wife, Elizabeth, who has been at my side since day one, and our two wonderful sons, Harrison and Jeremy. Without their encouragement and endless optimism, this book would have never seen the light of day.

Second, I must thank my colleague, Anne Trias, who has worked tirelessly with me over the last thirteen years and put countless hours into the development of this book.

And last, I would like to extend my gratitude to Keith and Kimberly Dunne, whose drive and dedication in getting this book over the line was unmatched.

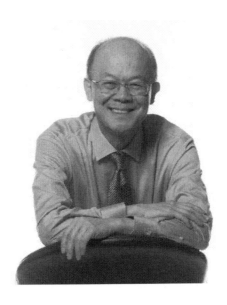

This book is written for *you* – the countless tens of thousands who are trying to live a healthier life.

Thank you so much for reading this book. I am very excited to share with you key pieces of information about an incredible form of vitamin E — tocotrienol. I will discuss its most important aspects to help you understand why it is the right and best type of vitamin E. And, I will explain how this form of E can help your body function well, and what conditions it can improve. It is my hope that once you've learned about tocotrienol, you will be able to make changes that will improve both your health and your life.

Dr. Barrie Tan
www.barrietan.com

WHAT IS INSIDE

Acknowledgments iii

INTRODUCTION vii

ONE: The Reason Behind My Research 1

TWO: A Love Affair with Tocotrienols................................7

THREE: The Importance of Cellular Health........................15

FOUR: All About E: An Introduction to the <u>Right</u> Vitamin E 19

FIVE: Difference and Interference 27

SIX: Documented Benefits and Functions of Tocotrienols 31

SEVEN: Conditions Tocotrienols Help Manage:
Part I: *Cardiovascular and Metabolic Health*.............................35

EIGHT: Conditions Tocotrienols Help Manage:
Part II: *Cancer, Bone, and Brain Health* 47

NINE: Conditions Tocotrienols Help Manage:
Part III: *All the Rest* 57

TEN: Protocol:
How to Get the Best Results from Tocotrienol.....................63

INTRODUCTION

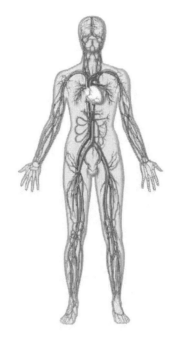

Arteries carry blood cells to import oxygen & nutrients **and to** export carbon dioxide & wastes **to**

38 trillion cells

Thirty-eight trillion. This is roughly the number of cells in your body.[1] With so many "moveable parts," a lot has to be in equilibrium and working right for you to be well — especially as you get older.

With the high cost of health care, more and more people are taking better care of themselves. So when you think about your heart, liver, brain, joints, and all those circulating fats, sugars, and cholesterol...think about the trillions of cells that make up you! And when you think about your cells, think about antioxidants, which are so important for cell health. And when you think about those important antioxidants, think about delta- and gamma- tocotrienols — the two most potent antioxidant and anti-inflammatory molecules in the vitamin E family – *with delta being the most potent*. It is these two that keep the moveable parts in check and in equilibrium. When that happens, your cells and arteries are happy. And so are you.

What exactly are tocotrienols?

Vitamin E is a family of eight separate but related molecules, including four tocopherols (delta, gamma, alpha, and beta) and four tocotrienols (also delta, gamma, alpha, and beta).

For many years, the scientific world, by fate, focused on only one part of vitamin E — its tocopherols. Why fate? It is an American affair. Tocopherol was discovered first, forty or fifty years before tocotrienol. Two UC Berkeley medical doctors found a substance in vegetables that helps gestation (bringing a fetus to full term). Almost 100 years ago they named it vitamin E.

It is only in the last ten years that the real star of the show, tocotrienol, started to shine — especially its delta and gamma molecules. Clinical studies show that tocotrienols, combined with a healthy lifestyle, do incredible things, including lowering lipids, reducing inflammation, protecting the liver, promoting bone health, killing cancer cells, and even increasing survival in cancer patients.

With the recent increase in studies on tocotrienols, researchers discovered that the "wrong" form of vitamin E (tocopherols) hindered the body's ability to absorb the "right" form (tocotrienols). A shocking turn of events! I'll explain more about this interference in Chapter 5.

But, before I dig into the science of it all, I will tell you about my exciting discovery of the antioxidant properties of the annatto plant, and how I was able to derive 100% tocotrienols (and only delta- and gamma- tocotrienols) from what I like to call my One Plant Wonder.

This is about to get exciting.

Really exciting.

ONE

The Reason Behind My Research

Just months before his doctor called me, Thomas had been close to death.

"This is incredible, Dr. Tan," he said. "Thomas has been taking annatto tocotrienol, and he is getting better. He was given a prognosis of only a few weeks to live. He's still alive after months!"

I was thrilled, of course. And, I remember taking a moment to soak in this news.

When I first started receiving calls from medical doctors and their patients telling me how much tocotrienol was helping, I felt amazed and thankful. After years and years of research, I was witnessing the bridge from lab to life appear, linking endless hours of reading and experiments, discussions and case studies, with real-world results. What a tremendous joy to hear how tocotrienols were making a positive difference in people's lives!

As a scientist, I am committed to well-designed research studies and clinical trials, and am driven by data-based conclusions. I also believe that studying plants and their color components for research's sake is valuable: the scientific enterprise of discovery, understanding how things work, uncovering hidden information, and figuring out novel approaches.

But I have to say what really gets me pumped up (and this has been true for more than forty years) is figuring out how those plants and colors benefit human health.

Remembering that phone call from Thomas's doctor still inspires me. It fuels my passion for understanding as much as I can about tocotrienols.

And the reports from doctors, patients, and researchers keep coming — often with results beyond what I ever imagined possible:

- Tumors shrinking
- Cholesterol numbers improving
- Heart conditions changing
- Cancer patients living longer
- Women's bones getting stronger
- Fatty liver improving and reversing
- Metabolic syndrome issues being assisted
- FD (familial dysautonomia) children experiencing cardiac stability
- Radiation protection possibilities
- Prostate benefits

I want to share with you just a few more examples of the letters and phone calls I have received:

Dear Dr. Tan,

I have to write to let you know how tocotrienol has helped my uncle with a very serious heart condition. We thought we had lost him forever, but since taking tocotrienol, he is experiencing a reversal and fantastic improvements. I am a doctor myself and had never heard about tocotrienol. Please send me more information, and I would love to meet you to discuss more.

_____

Dear Dr. Tan,

My 80-lb determined friend with Stage 4 breast cancer that had metastasized to her lymph nodes and liver refused chemotherapy because she wanted to fight this ugly disease in a healthier way. After taking 900 mg/day of tocotrienol, she noticed great results. Her doctor was skeptical at first. It has now been 6 months and she just texted me that she is, "Cancer Free!" She eats well and is taking other supplements. This is amazing!

_____

Dear Dr. Tan,

I have been reading about supplements that can help with healthy cholesterol levels. I have not done well on statin drugs and read that tocotrienol might help. I have been keeping close track of my numbers for the last two years, and I must let you know that my levels have greatly improved.

_____

Dear Dr. Tan,

I am an ophthalmologist and I have been a patient participating in a pancreatic cancer trial that used annatto tocotrienol. The trial has now ended, but I am still alive! Please let me know where I can purchase tocotrienol so that I may continue taking it.

―――――――――

Dear Dr. Tan,

I have lupus and my hands swell so badly at times that it is too painful to hold the steering wheel in my car. Even with shots, I have not been able to experience much change. Since taking tocotrienol, I have started to see the inflammation in my hands reduced.

―――――――――

Dear Dr. Tan,

My dog has arthritis and I love him so much. It hurts me to see him struggle. I decided to see what would happen if I gave him tocotrienol, and I want to let you know that it is helping with his ability to walk. Thank you so much!

―――――――――

Dear Dr. Tan,

Can you imagine what it is like to have a child who has never cried tears? That is a common experience for children with FD, a rare genetic neurologic disease. I had heard from other families whose children had been taking tocotrienol that they had started crying real tears. I want to let you know that today while out walking with my son, he mentioned that he cried while watching a movie. That was a walkstopper!

I have now opened many, many letters and received phone calls from all over the world. Each one moves me deeply, and I am completely energized, inspired, and humbled by the positive impact of tocotrienols on people's lives.

In the chapters ahead, I will continue to explain more about this incredible plant-based vitamin and how it can help you — as a powerful antioxidant for everyday health at the cellular level, and for numerous health conditions and concerns. Please read on!

TWO

A Love Affair with Tocotrienols

*I have been fortunate to discover the three major sources of
tocotrienols – rice, palm, and annatto.
These are still the commercially available sources today.*

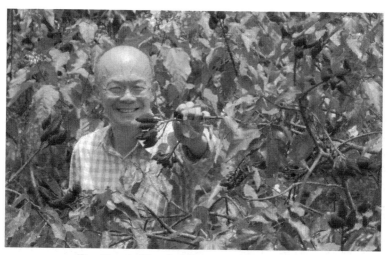

Dr. Barrie Tan holding an annatto plant

I have two loves in my life: my wife, Elizabeth, and tocotrienols.
A love affair with tocotrienol? What do you expect from a
researcher and scientist? But this passion led me to my fate:
discovery of the amazing antioxidant properties of the annatto,
a tropical plant that grows in South America.

Before I dive into this discovery, let me first tell you a little bit about me and how my unusual love affair began.

I earned my Bachelor of Science and a Ph.D. in chemistry at the University of Otago, New Zealand. Later, I became a professor at the University of Massachusetts at Amherst, first in chemistry, then in food science and nutrition.

My research included vitamin E, cholesterol and fats, prediabetes, diabetes, cancer and free radicals, along with lipid-soluble materials, such as carotenoids, CoQ10, and omega-3s.

In 1983, I was invited by a friend to visit a palm oil manufacturer in Malaysia, where I am originally from. Palm is known for having a large number of carotenes (brightly colored pigments important for photosynthesis), and I noticed that during manufacturing these orangey carotenoids were separated as a byproduct. I couldn't stop staring and wondering what might be the precise chemical components inside the crude oil.

On returning to the U.S., my curiosity drove me to begin extensive research on the oil. I noticed a light brownish portion that seemed to have high antioxidant properties; these were neither the fats nor the carotenes. My tests revealed results that were very close to those known for vitamin E tocopherols, but not exactly. Further research revealed the light brown material to be vitamin E of a different kind. What I found were tocotrienols! I started publishing these findings in 1986.

Several years later, my wife and I took a vacation to Phuket, Thailand. Just prior to leaving, I received an unexpected phone call from a counselor to one of the princes of Thailand. He had heard about my background in carotenoids, and wished to set up a meeting between the prince and me to discuss a research and development proposal. The prince wanted to sponsor research dedicated to discovering new plant-based nutraceuticals.

A company was formed and in it we discovered that rice, too, was a source of tocotrienols.

In the early 1990s, I took a break from vitamin E and became interested in the work being done by Dr. Johanna Seddon, a renowned ophthalmologist and retina specialist. Dr. Seddon discovered that at the back of the retina are levels of lutein and zeaxanthin that help combat macular degeneration.

I was told that if I went to South America, I would find a giant marigold flower about the size of an orange, and I could extract lutein and zeaxanthin from its petals. So, with excitement, I went to South America to find a flower that could potentially help many people with age-related macular degeneration.

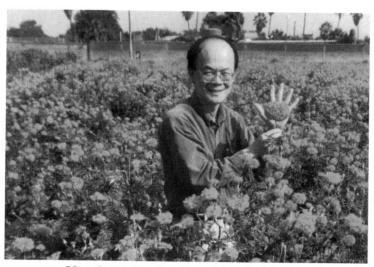

Here I am, standing in a field of marigolds

As you can see from the photo above, I found my giant marigold! But, as chance would have it, while holding this bright marigold blossom, I noticed an annatto plant just thirty feet away. I was stunned by the beauty of the plant. When the fruit pod opened, I only saw seeds, no flesh. I rubbed it, and an intense red oil coated my hand. There is a reason the British nicknamed this the "lipstick plant." But I call it my One Plant Wonder.

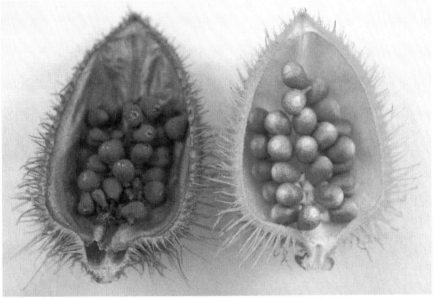

The seeds of the annatto plant

For a long minute I stood transfixed, staring at the red seeds. How could the beautiful red color possibly still be so strong? Without any flesh to protect them, the seeds were directly exposed to the sun and air. The intense red-to-maroon colored seeds should have been turning brown, but they were not. I wondered what was inside protecting the seeds? I suspected that there must be a very powerful antioxidant that the annatto plant made to protect its carotenoids. "It must be polyphenols,"

I thought. They are powerful antioxidants and are ubiquitous in the plant kingdom.

FUN FACT

The red oil from the annatto seed is used as a natural coloring in cheeses, like cheddar, Gloucester, and Red Leicester. You can also find it in many other foods, including ice cream, meats, crackers, seasonings, salad dressings, tortilla chips, and even mac & cheese.

When I returned to the states, I showed this plant to John Foley, my good friend and lab chemist at the time. We immediately started to decipher what was in the annatto seeds that kept the carotene pigment red. When the results emerged, I was shocked — it was vitamin E. I was further shocked to learn that it only contained tocotrienols. And most shocked when I realized it only contained delta- and gamma-tocotrienols!

That, for me, was one of my happiest and most unexpected moments as a scientist.

Delta and gamma are the most potent tocotrienols; alpha comes in third, with beta at the rear. So imagine finding a plant that has just delta and gamma. The American Chemical Society currently has fifty million unique chemicals registered in their database[2] — this was a true needle-in-the-haystack experience!

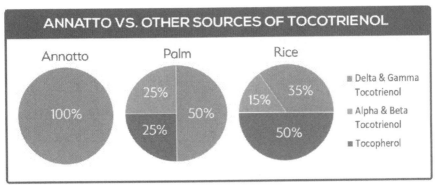

Figure 1: Sources of Tocotrienol

As you now know, I discovered the three major sources of tocotrienols: palm oil c. 1984, rice c. 1995, and annatto c. 1999. Palm oil has 50% delta- and gamma-tocotrienols, rice has 35% delta- and gamma-tocotrienols, and annatto has 100% delta- and gamma-tocotrienol. Additionally, palm and rice sources contain 25 to 50% tocopherol; annatto has none (see Figure 1).

In 1998, with the help of my wife, I started a natural health R&D company called American River Nutrition, which is where I developed the first-ever tocopherol-free tocotrienol product extracted from annatto. The product, DeltaGold®, was released to the nutritional and natural health care industry in 2005 and is currently an ingredient in many major brands.

During this time, tocotrienols were starting to gain attention for their health benefits. I decided to focus on an earth-friendly and more efficient way to extract the tocotrienols, particularly from annatto.

You see, tocotrienols exist at low levels in nature, so it was important to find an easier, cost-effective way to extract this priceless gem. I was awarded the first-ever annatto patent for a unique extraction technique in 2002. This technique allowed us to extract DeltaGold® without using harsh or synthetic chemicals, petrochemicals, or solvents — so nothing similar to those that are commonly used in extraction. It is purely a physical and evaporative technique, making DeltaGold® truly 100% natural!

Today I am dedicated to in-depth research for developing phytonutrients to reduce and slow chronic disorders that plague many of us as we age.

THREE

The Importance of Cellular Health

Tocotrienols fight off free radicals and keep your cell membranes strong and protected.

"The more you know, the more you grow." That's an old saying that rings true when it comes to understanding cellular health. In this chapter, I will provide you with an introduction to cell membranes, free radicals, and how antioxidants like tocotrienols help maintain a healthy lifestyle. Knowing this information will help you appreciate the way vitamins and supplements support overall health.

The Cell Membrane

It is essential to understand what the cell membrane is and why we need it to be healthy.

A cell membrane is a thin casing that surrounds the cell. Its wall-like function is to protect the cell by allowing certain substances in while keeping others out.

Phospholipids (fatty acids), cholesterol, and a small amount of protein make up most of the cell membrane. Phospholipids create a lipid bilayer (a universal two-layered structure of fat cells) while proteins help move selective molecules in and out of this bilayer. This arrangement is important, because it allows for essential molecules such as water, oxygen, and carbon dioxide to cross the membrane while blocking other larger and potentially harmful substances.

Due to the fact that a cell's membrane is made of unstable fatty acids and often unsaturated fats (such as omega-3s), it needs a lot of protection from oxidation and free-floating toxins and pollutants that roam throughout the body.

This is where tocotrienols come in (especially delta-tocotrienol). They help maintain membrane integrity to better protect cellular functions.

Free Radicals

Next, let's learn about free radicals, the bullies on the block. Free radicals are overcharged oxygen molecules that have become unstable. Stress, pollutants, smoking, bad foods, bad fats, too much exposure to ultraviolet rays from the sun — all things that can cause our bodies to produce these overcharged oxygen radicals.

Because free radicals are unstable, they attack and steal electrons from stable molecules within healthy cells in an attempt to stabilize themselves. This damages the cells. In a micro picture, damaged cells lead to cell dysfunction and death. In a macro picture, damaged cells lead to premature aging and disease.

However, free radicals are still important for a healthy life. They are needed to kill invading pathogens, like those that might land on an open wound. It sounds like a contradiction, doesn't it? It is only when they get out of control that the trouble begins. While we don't want to wipe out free radicals completely, we also need to keep them at a low level, activated only when an acute need arises — for example, a bacterial infection. This is where antioxidants come in!

Antioxidants

Simply put, antioxidants are molecules in cells that typically come from nutrients, the most common being vitamins A, C, E, and the minerals selenium and zinc. When a free radical attacks a healthy cell to get its missing electron, the antioxidant molecule attached to that cell gives the free radical its own electron without destabilizing the cell.

A few other well-known antioxidants are resveratrol, curcumin, astaxanthin, lutein, coenzyme Q10 (CoQ10), and of course, tocotrienols. Tocotrienols in particular are well suited to protect the cell membrane because their perfect fit into the lipid bilayer allows them to better protect the lipids within this bilayer from oxidation.

Let's put this all together

Imagine you have just taken a supplement of annatto tocotrienol. Your small intestine soon absorbs this antioxidant through its walls and pushes it out into your lymph and then into your bloodstream. The delta- and gamma-tocotrienols spread out and attach themselves to a variety of cell membranes throughout your body and then start patrolling for free radicals. As soon as they sense one closing in (meaning the free radical attaches to a fatty acid in the cell wall), the tocotrienol molecule releases an electron which re-attaches to the free radical, making the damaged (oxidized) fatty acid in the cell wall whole again. The free radical is stable again and leaves the cell. Put simply, the tocotrienol removes the aberrant oxygen from the fatty acid.

It is amazing what the body can do, and even more amazing what tocotrienol can do to help the body ward off unwanted advances of oxygen.

FOUR

All About E: An Introduction to the <u>Right</u> Vitamin E

It took 42 years for the scientific community to discover that tocotrienols are a part of vitamin E.

The aim of this chapter is to help you understand vitamin E as a whole, as well as appreciate its individual parts. In order to do this, I will first introduce you to the structure of vitamin E, followed by a brief overview of its history before wrapping up with an attempt to untangle the knot of false claims that surround this great nutrient.

Structure of Vitamin E

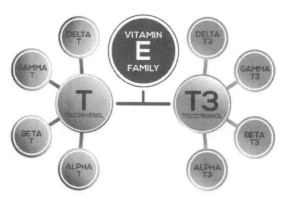

Figure 2: Structure of vitamin E

As I mentioned in the introduction, vitamin E is a family of eight separate but related fat-soluble molecules. These are split into two groups, tocopherols and tocotrienols. Each group contains four molecules: a delta, gamma, alpha, and beta form (see Figure 2).

Having healthy fats and lipids in your diet is important because they help your cells better absorb the fat-soluble tocotrienols and store them in your body for future use. We get our healthy fats from sources like nuts and fish. And what about lipids? Lipids are molecules that make up the structure of cells. Examples of lipids are oils, cholesterol, specialized proteins, lipid vitamins, and nutrients.

You have probably already heard about vitamin E, and most likely, you're familiar with its most publicized element: alpha-tocopherol. This form of vitamin E is being reassessed because recent research has revealed its inferior — and even potentially harmful — effects. In other words, alpha-tocopherol benefits have been greatly overrated.

I wrote this book because I wanted to increase awareness of the very powerful, yet lesser-known benefits of the *right* form of vitamin E – annatto tocotrienol (a combination of both delta- and gamma-tocotrienol).

A Brief History of Vitamin E

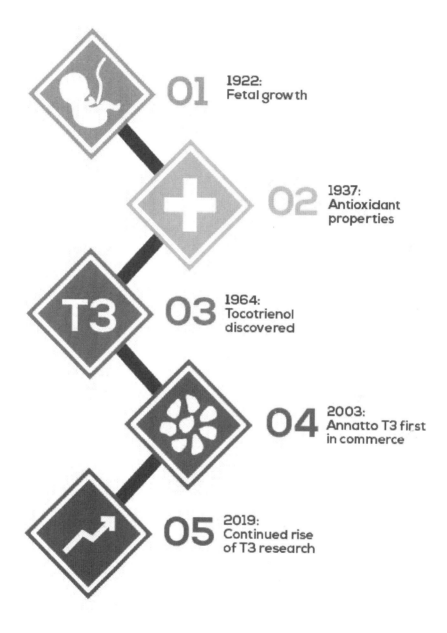

01 1922:
Fetal growth

02 1937:
Antioxidant
properties

03 1964:
Tocotrienol
discovered

04 2003:
Annatto T3 first
in commerce

05 2019:
Continued rise
of T3 research

Vitamin E was discovered in 1922 by two University of California physicians, Herbert McLean Evans and Katharine

Scott Bishop, as a vital nutrient to prevent birth defects. They were experimenting with fertility in rats when they came across a compound in wheat germ that allowed the pregnant female rats to reach full term. Evans named the molecules "tocopherol," from the Greek words "τόκος" [birth], and "φέρειν" [to bear or carry], meaning in sum "to carry a pregnancy." For a time, the unknown component was termed vitamin X and the "anti-sterility factor."

It was fifteen years before the next use for vitamin E was brought to light. In 1937, two scientists, H.S. Olcott & O.H Emerson, discovered that tocopherols contained antioxidant properties.[3]

So far, we have only talked about tocopherols. It wasn't until 1964 that tocotrienols were discovered — and that was by accident! When first seen by chromatography, tocotrienols looked like shadows on a piece of paper — almost like tocopherols' shadows. They were mistakenly classified as new tocopherols. *This is why there is so much information on tocopherols and so little on tocotrienols.* Another reason tocotrienols are not as well-known is because there are numerous tocopherol-rich sources available and only a limited number of tocotrienol-rich sources.

The number of studies conducted on tocotrienols during this time was also scarce because many of the initial studies were undertaken using palm oil (the first-known commercial source of tocotrienol). Palm oil contains a high percentage of alpha-tocopherol, which actually interferes with the absorption of tocotrienols in the body. I remember being surprised to see more and more researchers noticing the blocking effect of tocopherol, which kept tocotrienols from performing at their best.

This use of palm oil lowered the effectiveness of tocotrienols used in these trials and discouraged further research. In the next chapter, I will go into more depth on the matter of alpha-tocopherol interference.

During the 1980s and into the 1990s, research uncovered that the two most potent vitamin E compounds were delta- and gamma-tocotrienols. The alpha-tocotrienol compound was a distant third, with beta-tocotrienol being the least potent. When combined, delta and gamma worked even better.

The next big breakthrough for vitamin E was one of my own — the discovery of annatto tocotrienol. As mentioned earlier, in 2005 I launched DeltaGold® into the market, a new vitamin E product that contains a whopping 90% delta-tocotrienol.

To this day, hundreds of research studies on tocotrienols for chronic issues are being conducted. Many of these studies are public records at the U.S. National Library of Medicine-National Institutes of Health at www.PubMed.gov. In previous decades, tocopherol research dwarfed tocotrienol studies. Today, it is the reverse (see Figure 3).

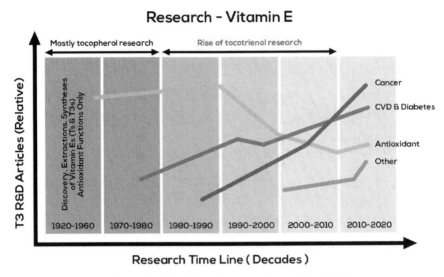

Figure 3: Timeline of research on vitamin E

"Vitamin E Does Not Work"

In the last ten to twenty years there has been a lot of negative news surrounding the benefits of vitamin E. For example, *"Vitamin E does not work,"* or *"Vitamin E may be harmful to your health."* How is this so, and are these claims true?

Many of the studies behind these claims used alpha-tocopherol exclusively, and others used synthetic alpha-tocopherol, often in excessive amounts. None used tocotrienol. At best, these trials failed; at worst, they may have produced harm. This caused tocopherol supplementation to sit uncomfortably with many consumers.

The original vitamin E measurement placed an inordinate emphasis on alpha-tocopherol. Vitamin E's value was its ability to prevent fetal resorption (or to bring a fetus to full term). Such activity was given a measurement, or currency, International Units (IU), and was assigned as per the table below.

Compound	Weight/Mass	Equivalent IU measurement
alpha-tocopherol	10 mg	10 IU
beta-tocopherol	10 mg	5 IU
gamma-tocopherol	10 mg	1 IU
alpha-tocotrienol	10 mg	5 IU
delta-tocopherol beta-tocotrienol gamma-tocotrienol delta-tocotrienol	10 mg	0 IU or Unkown

Seeing the monetizable IU currency of alpha-tocopherol, the industry converted all tocopherols to alpha-tocopherol. For example, the most common soy mixed tocopherols (typically containing 15% alpha-tocopherol and 85% gamma- and delta-tocopherols) are chemically converted to only alpha-tocopherol.

The IU currency for vitamin E is a misguided and useless measure, and the FDA has since scrapped its use. All vitamin E tocopherols and tocotrienols are now labeled in milligrams (mgs). This further supports the movement away from alpha-tocopherol.

Conclusion

Vitamin E has had its share of ups and downs in the past, but I promise you the best is yet to come. There has been an influx of studies and research on tocotrienols that show great advances for health and I am excited to see what happens next. The *right* form of vitamin E is now available. It is safe, 100% natural, and a great companion to a healthy lifestyle.

FIVE

Difference and Interference

Tocotrienols are 40-60 times more potent than tocopherols.

I have been promising to talk in more depth about tocotrienols, tocopherols, and how they interact, so here we go! I have provided below the three key chemical and structural differences between the two molecules, followed by an understanding of how they interact.

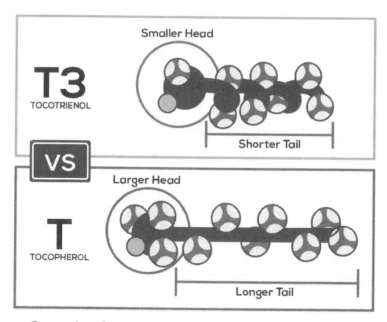

Comparison between tocotrienol and tocopherol molecules

Key Differences

#1: Tocotrienols have shorter tails that do not anchor deeply into the cell membrane. This allows them to move around the cell membrane faster — *fifty times faster!* — and therefore intercept free radicals more easily. Tocopherols, on the other hand, have longer tails, anchor deeply into the cell membranes, and hence move more slowly to intercept free radicals. If vitamin Es were cell phones, tocopherols would be 1G and tocotrienols would be 50G.

From a study conducted by Dr. Lester Packer, we know that tocotrienols are considerably more potent than tocopherols as an antioxidant. Packer observed that tocotrienols were spinning around the cells much faster than the tocopherols. Because of this, he theorized that tocotrienols are forty to sixty times better at giving one of their electrons to the invading free radicals and thereby repairing damage to the lipids on the membranes.[4]

#2: Tocotrienols have smaller heads and delta-tocotrienol has the smallest. The smaller heads on tocotrienols allow them to squeeze into parts of the cell easier than tocopherols can. This provides tocotrienols wider access to membranes and increases their ability to capture more free radicals than tocopherols can.

#3: Tocotrienols have unsaturated tails, tocopherols have saturated tails. This means that tocotrienols are unique in that they have three double bonds in their tails whereas tocopherols do not. This also means that tocotrienols can provide more lipid oxidation protection because of their superior bioavailability to cell membranes. The same is true for cancer cells: tocotrienol's bioavailability allows it to kill cancer cells. This is remarkable.

Interference

A crucial concept to grasp when discussing vitamin E is the interference that occurs when we have too much alpha-tocopherol in our system.

Alpha-tocopherol is unique because it has an alpha-TTP (alpha-tocopherol transfer protein) as well as the ability to protect LDL from oxidation. Think of the transfer protein as a passport that allows alpha-tocopherol to gain admittance and enter the bloodstream. A typical American diet provides all the alpha-tocopherol we need for it to do this job.

The interference occurs when we have too much alpha-tocopherol in our system (for example, taking alpha-tocopherol as a supplement). Our passageways become filled with these molecules that, because they have the right of way, impede tocotrienols from absorption and entry into the bloodstream.

So how much alpha-tocopherol is too much? Good question! In a healthy diet, it is expected we consume about 10-15 mgs of tocopherols per day. Such amounts do not present any interference to tocotrienols.

There are *no other known contraindications with tocotrienol outside of alpha-tocopherol.* It is synergistic with vitamin C and mixes well with other lipid (fat) nutrients such as carotenoids, fish oil, and CoQ10.

Conclusion

Each day it is becoming increasingly understood that tocotrienols (especially delta-tocotrienols) are the right form of vitamin E. Well in excess of 100 studies and clinical trials have shown the surprising benefits of tocotrienols – without any known side effects.

SIX

Documented Benefits and Functions of Tocotrienols

I am fully convinced of the benefits of tocotrienols.

I am excited and confident about the potential of this natural supplement. Below is a summary of the benefits I have ascertained with the use of DeltaGold® (annatto tocotrienol):

- **Helps Maintain a Healthy Brain for Healthy Aging**
  Tocotrienols, in addition to a healthy lifestyle, may help keep you sharp and contribute to better brain health.[5] In fact, population-based studies conducted by the Karolinska Institute showed that higher levels of vitamin E tocopherols and tocotrienols in elderly subjects were associated with a lower risk of cognitive impairment and Alzheimer's disease. [6-9]

- **Helps Maintain a Healthy Blood Sugar Level**
  We need a healthy amount of blood sugar (glucose) to give our cells and organs energy. Glucose is helping you read this book with ease and understanding because blood sugar also energizes your brain cells. Keeping normal blood levels is an important goal throughout life.

- **Helps Maintain Healthy Cells**
  Remember: when you think of your health, think of your cells. We have thirty-eight *trillion* of them! Your cells are the bottom line for all-around health and, as you learned in Chapter 3, tocotrienols play an important part in maintaining cellular health. This includes preventing cells from going rancid and aberrant. Tocotrienols could potentially turn "rancid" and "aberrant" cells back to normal.

- **Keeps Cardiovascular Health and Cholesterol Levels in Check**
  Tocotrienols are nutrients that help give you peace of mind, because they (along with a healthy lifestyle) help keep your healthy lipids in check and nurture your cardiovascular system.

- **Reverses Metabolic and Liver Maladies**
  The liver performs more than 500 essential functions, and keeping it healthy cannot be taken for granted. A fatty liver makes an unhealthy liver. When you lower your risk for metabolic syndrome and fatty liver maladies, you raise your hope for healthier aging for years to come.

- **Maintains Healthy Bones**
  Where would you be without a good, strong skeleton? Not very far! In many studies delta- and gamma-tocotrienols have already shown promise for strengthening bones, including bones in post-menopausal women with osteopenia.[10-12]

- **Radiation Protection**

  While radiation exposure does not affect everyone, it is still a big concern because radiation can stick around for a long time. For those who are affected, tocotrienols help protect sensitive cells from destructive ionizing radiation.

- **Keeps Inflammation at Bay**

  What would your day be like if your inflammation wasn't as bad? Tocotrienols calm your cells and provide relief from inflammation that could later turn into chronic health issues.

- **Upgrades All Cells to Lipid Antioxidant Protection**

  This means your cells are better protected, including your heart, brain, prostate, breasts, and especially your liver and fat pad. Talk about having better peace of mind. Upgrades to your computer operating system are often a pain, but for your cells there is a definite upside.

SEVEN

Conditions Tocotrienols Help Manage: Part I

Cardiovascular and Metabolic Health

Now that you have a good understanding of tocotrienols (especially the delta and gamma ones), I can move on to discuss the many conditions they have shown to help manage.

I feel safe in assuming that you would not be reading this book if you, or someone you know, did not have a health problem you wanted to solve, or help solve. And I'm confident you understand that tocotrienols cannot solve all your problems on their own — they are not a silver bullet (does such a thing even exist?).

So, if you really want to improve your health, you have to invest in more than just taking supplements. Engaging in more exercise and physical activity, getting more and better sleep, and eating right are just a few of the things you already know are important. This advice has been around for a long time and with good reason. Even small changes will improve your health and well-being, especially for individuals with poor cardiovascular and metabolic health. Please read on to see how tocotrienols, in tandem with a healthy lifestyle, can really jump-start your recovery.

Chronic Inflammation

The traditional view of cardiovascular disease associates elevated cholesterol with clogged arteries. Surprisingly, half of patients presenting with heart attacks have normal cholesterol levels. Today, it is well-known that inflammation acts as cholesterol's partner in crime in cardiovascular disease progression by recruiting white blood cells to damaged arteries, causing them to stick and initiate a "clogged-pipe" at the plaque site.

Tocotrienols have been shown to have potent ability to reduce inflammation and new research is focused on this effect. These studies demonstrate that alpha-, gamma-, and delta-tocotrienols strongly inhibit the inflammatory response such as NF kappaB (NFkB) and tumor necrosis factor-a (TNF-a), along with a lot of inflammation "handlers".

Two clinical studies on tocotrienol showed the supplement's impressive ability to deliver a one-two punch to elevated cholesterol levels and inflammation.[13,14] It is encouraging to see how delta-tocotrienol, in particular, works to calm inflammation levels.

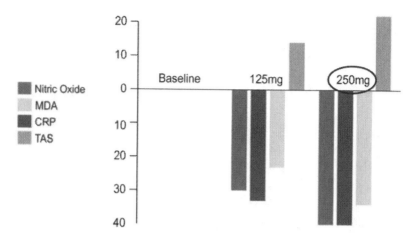

Phase duration (4wk) and washout (2wk)

Figure 4: Results of a trial on cholesterol & inflammation in hypercholesterolemic patients

Among the most notable biomarkers to be affected by a 250 mg tocotrienol daily dosage were C-reactive protein (CRP; a predictor for chronic inflammation), nitric oxide (NO), and malondialdehyde (MDA), with decreases of 40%, 40%, and 34%, respectively (see Figure 4).

Total antioxidant status (TAS), on the other hand, increased by 22%. This suggests delta-tocotrienol potentiates endogenous antioxidants. Several inflammatory cytokines and microRNAs were found to be modulated by tocotrienol treatment, suggesting more favorable outcomes in cardiovascular and aging diseases with supplement use.

When combined with other anti-inflammatory ingredients, tocotrienols showed synergistic efficacy. Two clinical studies show that delta-tocotrienol in combination with antioxidant polyphenols curb inflammation and manage dyslipidemia.[15,16]

One of the placebo-controlled studies was conducted in two groups of elderly subjects, one with normal and the other with elevated lipid levels. The product formulation was composed of 50 mg delta-tocotrienol from annatto (as found in DeltaGold®), along with a B-vitamin (niacin), and polyphenols. In both groups, supplementation led to a significant drop in CRP and γ-glutamyl transferase (a predictor for non-fatal myocardial infarction and fatal coronary heart disease), while increasing total antioxidant status, a measure of the body's capacity to counteract reactive oxygen species.

In the hypercholesterolemic group, LDL cholesterol (20-28%) and triglycerides (11-18%) also dropped. C-reactive protein dropped in healthy elderly (21-29%) as well as lipidemic elderly (31-48%), as did γ-glutamyl transferase (14-20%). Notably, there were no adverse effects associated with the six-week supplementation period.[15,16]

What does all this mean for you? Tocotrienols' proven ability to reduce inflammation can help prevent many associated diseases and chronic conditions, improving your overall health.

High Cholesterol

As you read earlier, tocotrienol and tocopherol molecules are structurally different. Tocotrienols have a shorter tail with double bonds. These double bonds help reduce the activity of the enzyme that controls the production of cholesterol, which is the same enzyme targeted by statin drugs. This enzyme is called 3-hydroxy-3-methylglutaryl coenzyme A reductase (HMG-CoAR). But tocotrienol and statins work differently on this enzyme.

Tocotrienols dial down cholesterol synthesis whereas statins shut down cholesterol synthesis. This is why statins are referred to as an "indiscriminate cholesterol reducer." Tocotrienols are a "discriminate cholesterol reducer."[17-19]

In addition, only gamma- and delta-tocotrienols stimulated the degradation of the HMG-CoAR, shown in 1992 and repeated fifteen years later in 2006.[17,19]

In another study, researchers wanted to know how to lower the fat in blood (triglycerides) using tocotrienols.

They first conducted tests in cell cultures and mice with high cholesterol and triglyceride levels. They discovered that tocotrienols reduce genes' ability to enable triglyceride production. It is thought that tocotrienols directly regulate triglyceride synthesis in the body, thus helping to lower excess fat in the blood.

They also discovered that tocotrienols help reduce VLDL, which is another type of fat related to triglycerides that can also lead to strokes and heart attacks.

The animal portion of this study showed that treatment with tocotrienols significantly reduced the fat level in the blood by 19% and cholesterol by 28%.[20]

Impressed by these results, the research group turned to human studies. They gave healthy men and women 120 mg gamma- and delta-tocotrienols per day for an eight-week trial. Not only did the subjects' fat levels in their blood drop by 28%, the triglyceride-related VLDL (bad cholesterol) trended down by 13%.[20]

If that weren't enough, tocotrienols also block the processing of a certain protein that helps control the LDL receptor (the receptor that helps keep your cholesterol in circulation). All these reduce fat in your blood, which is important in prediabetic and diabetic conditions. The other vitamin E molecules do not block this process or hinder it in any way. Only gamma- and delta-tocotrienols do this.[19]

Cardiovascular Disease

Chronic inflammation is the "perpetual flame" of many diseases, including cardiovascular disease. One of the ways it flares up is when the immune system attacks LDL ("bad" cholesterol) that is attached to arterial walls. Ongoing inflammation eventually damages the arteries. This can create more oxidized materials just inside the artery walls (called plaques) and can cause them to rupture or burst.

In fact, doctors now use a test for inflammation called CRP (a "shout-out" stress protein produced in the liver) to assess a person's risk of heart attack, given the close association between inflammation and heart disease.

In several trials, tocotrienols have demonstrated their ability to affect high cholesterol levels, hinder the oxidation of fat, quell inflammation, and subsequently reduce the "velcro effect" on artery walls.[13,14]

In vitro studies (experiments or procedures that are done outside of the body, such as in a test tube or laboratory dish) have found that tocotrienols resist oxidation to LDL cholesterol[21], which is thought to be a crucial initiating step for atherosclerosis. Atherosclerosis is a common disorder that occurs when fat, cholesterol, calcium, and other rancid material build up in the walls of arteries and form plaques. On the contrary, many may not know, alpha-tocopherol can oxidize LDL cholesterol.[22]

Free radicals and inflammation can lead to diabetes, obesity, and fatty liver for many people, especially when they attack repeatedly and over time. Taking antioxidants, along with having a healthier lifestyle, are a successful shield to these oxidative and inflammatory attacks.

Metabolic Syndrome (MetS)

Metabolic syndrome (MetS) is a cluster of conditions like moderately high blood sugar, high fat, high cholesterol, and high blood pressure that all happen together, and can increase your risk for heart disease, stroke, and diabetes.

In one study on the effect of tocotrienols on MetS, researchers fed rats a high carb, high fat diet to induce obesity with accompanying cardiac remodeling, insulin resistance, hypertension, and fatty liver. The animals then received oral alpha-tocopherol, alpha-, gamma-, or delta-tocotrienols at 85 mg per day, corresponding to a 60 kg human dose of ~800 mg per day. Results showed that, while all these vitamin E molecules reduced the number of inflammatory cells in the heart, only delta- and gamma-tocotrienols improved cardiovascular function and systolic blood pressure.

Furthermore, only delta-tocotrienol affected important markers of MetS and diabetes in three ways: 1. By helping the body create and process the glucose better; 2. By improving insulin sensitivity; and, 3. By reducing lipids (a form of fat) and abdominal fat. All this resulted in a reduction in organ inflammation, especially in the heart, liver, and abdominal fat.[23]

A similar study confirmed these results by studying mice that were fed a high fat diet. The researchers examined the effects of stored fat around connective tissues like cartilage, bone, blood, and bone marrow.

The approximate human equivalent of tocotrienols given to the mice was 160-640 mg per day for 14 weeks, at which point improvements in glucose tolerance along with reduced fat levels in the liver and blood were observed. In addition, the size of the fat cells and liver tissues were reduced, resulting in overall improved health of the fat and of the liver.[24]

Two closely-related groups of research further added to this MetS study using tocotrienols. One group separately looked at delta and gamma, and these tocotrienols attenuated "nascent flames" — called inflammasomes — of macrophages that protected chronic metabolic diseases.[25] The other research group looked at the impact of tocotrienols with alpha-tocopherol removed. They found that tocopherol-free rice bran tocotrienol (RBT3) had anti-lipidemic effects, reducing cholesterol (15%) and triglycerides (28%) simultaneously.[26]

So, across three continents, several independent studies demonstrated that delta and gamma do the same job to protect fat and the liver. That's great!

So what does all this mean for you and your health? Having more than one chronic condition increases your chances of developing a disease or suffering a heart attack or stroke. Because studies show that delta- and gamma-tocotrienols lower high risk factors for many diseases and conditions, they can have a broad and beneficial effect on your overall health.

Nonalcoholic Fatty Liver Disease (NAFLD)

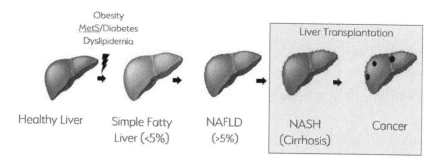

Stages of liver disease

Nonalcoholic fatty liver disease, or NAFLD is the new name for liver problems. NAFLD happens when there is too much fat stored in the liver cells. This condition is not related to alcohol consumption and is mostly caused by diet. The staggering reality is that eighty to one hundred million Americans have this disease.[27,28]

Nonalcoholic steatohepatitis (NASH), which is a more serious form of the disease, is indicated by liver inflammation and fibrosis. This may result in scarred tissues and irreversible damage. This damage is similar to the damage caused by overdrinking, but those affected are not drinkers. NASH can turn to cirrhosis and liver failure.

A randomized, double-blind, placebo-controlled study was conducted in seventy-one patients having ultrasound-proven fatty liver disease. They were given either 300 mg of tocotrienols twice a day or a placebo for twelve weeks.

Out of seventy-one patients, sixty-four of them — thirty-one in the tocotrienol group and thirty-three in the placebo group — completed the study. After twelve weeks, tocotrienols showed a greater effect than the placebo by enhancing liver function.

Significant improvements were also shown in stress reduction related to the liver. CRP and MDA — both markers of inflammation and fat oxidation — decreased by 18% and 14% after three months, respectively. Tocotrienols were considered a safe natural aid for excess inflammation and free radicals in patients with NAFLD.

In addition, a significant decrease of fat in the blood showed reduced inflammation that was consistent with the results of previous clinical trials conducted with DeltaGold® for people with an excess of cholesterol in their blood and liver. The fatty liver index score (a measure of fat in liver storage) decreased by 11%.

What made this study even more remarkable, especially for the patients, is that the tocotrienol-supplemented group lost an average of 9.7 pounds, with a resultant decrease in BMI and waistline. [29]

What this means for you is that when your liver is less "fatty," it can better filter out the (environmental) toxins in your body and break down fats and make proteins, allowing it to more efficiently and effectively perform its over five hundred biological functions. With a better functioning liver, your overall health will improve.

Diabetes and Prediabetes

About 10% of the US population has diabetes, so learning more about how tocotrienols can help lower the risk factor and/or manage this disease is extremely important. Here you will discover the connection between tocotrienols, diabetes, and PPAR alpha.

PPAR alpha, also known as peroxisome proliferator-activated receptor alpha, is important in regulating lipid metabolism in the liver. Activation of PPAR alpha can help control hypertriglyceridemia (elevated blood triglycerides), which is one of the hallmarks of metabolic syndrome.

Tocotrienols were shown to activate PPAR alpha, which helps control the genes that are involved with burning fatty acids for fuel. PPAR alpha activated by tocotrienols also improved blood glucose and insulin sensitivity. These are important aspects of metabolism for lowering triglycerides and raising blood sugar metabolism.[30]

Gamma- and delta-tocotrienols are effective for lowering triglycerides by restraining genes that start triglyceride production. Triglycerides are a type of fat or lipid found in your blood. The triglycerides you eat or that are converted inside your body are sent to fat cells where they are stored and often show up as what we fondly call a "love handle." Hormones regulate the release of triglycerides from fat tissue so they meet your body's needs for energy between meals.

High levels of these fats are closely linked to an increased risk of heart attacks, strokes, Alzheimer's disease, atherosclerosis, diabetes, and other chronic ills. Scientists found that after two months of supplementation, gamma- and delta-tocotrienols were effective in lowering triglyceride levels by 28% in the blood of human subjects,[20] and by 10% in MetS patients with NAFLD.[29]

It is known that omega-3 fish oil can also lower triglycerides, with one big difference: the amount of tocotrienol needed to do the same task is about 10x lower. Nevertheless, it makes good sense to take delta-tocotrienol and omega-3 together.

EIGHT

Conditions Tocotrienols Help Manage: Part II

Cancer, Bone, and Brain Health

As I begin this next section, I want to highlight again how much exercise can't be over emphasized. Taking a brisk 20-30 minute walk every day can make a difference. Taking the stairs instead of the elevator and standing more at your desk rather than sitting all day are surprisingly proven ways to lower your risk. I try not to sit for more than one hour at a time. If you haven't done so already, make a pledge to yourself to do more than enjoy a healthier diet, commit to increasing how much you move each day.

Cancer

In addition to their superior antioxidant power and showing promise for reducing the formation of blood clots, tocotrienols have shown consistent anti-tumor benefits. Some researchers attribute these anti-cancer effects to tocotrienols' antioxidant activity, HMG-CoAR inhibition,[31] and vascular endothelial growth factor (VEGF) inhibition.[32] VEGF is a signal protein produced by your cells to stimulate the formation of blood vessels.[33]

Tocotrienols, *not tocopherols*, have repeatedly been shown to hinder the rapid multiplying of cancer cells. Cells with the greatest degree of malignancy are most sensitive to the action of tocotrienols. In all cases, delta- and gamma-tocotrienols were the two most potent vitamin E molecules to inhibit cancer growth. There are many possible modes of action for cancer kill by tocotrienols for a wide range of different types of cancers. One such type is breast cancer. Tocotrienol has been shown to hinder the rapid growth of breast cancer cells while alpha-tocopherol had no effect.[34]

Did you know that estrogen may send signals to breast cancer cells that may increase their growth? Another study found that tocotrienols inhibit this, with gamma- and delta-tocotrienols being the most potent.[35]

DID YOU KNOW?

Of all the tocopherol and tocotrienol molecules, only delta and gamma attach to tumors, and, by doing so, help kill them. They do not harm normal cells and they have a penchant for aberrant ones.

Because gamma- and delta-tocotrienols were shown — in reproducible tests — to slow down or, in some cases, prevent cancer, tocotrienols in their purest natural form should be included during cancer treatment. A clinical trial using a tocopherol and tocotrienol mixture in breast cancer patients did not work and it was therefore indicated that pure gamma-tocotrienol should be used instead to avoid tocopherol interference issues. Such a trial, however, has not materialized.

As mentioned earlier, tocotrienols help reduce the activity of HMG-CoAR. More specifically, the gamma-tocotrienol molecule was found to be responsible for slowing down the cholesterol production in the liver by reducing the HMG-CoAR enzyme.

While your liver uses this HMG-CoAR cholesterol-production pathway to produce LDL cholesterol for your entire body, every cell in your body also uses the same pathway to produce this small waxy lipid that is vital for maintaining the health and survival of any cell.

In situations of cancer, however...

...this pathway is hijacked and used by cancer cells to spread the produced cholesterol throughout the tumor, fueling its growth. Researchers realized that the tocotrienols in the liver and healthy cells would be very different inside cancer cells — tocotrienols directly stymied aberrant HMG-CoAR activity (in cancer) from synthesizing cholesterol.[36] This is a highly specific function of tocotrienol.

In other words, tocotrienols have a remarkable ability to tell the difference between healthy cells and cancer cells. In the case of cancer, tocotrienols could seriously weaken the cancer cells' multiplying and proliferation ability. Statins can also kill cancer this way, but the dose required to kill cancer in humans is prohibitively high and associated with serious side effects.[37]

Tocotrienols have also been shown to help chemo drugs work much better, especially in resistant and recurring cancer cells. Scientists and oncologists call this "chemosensitization."

For breast and skin cancers, delta- and gamma-tocotrienols contain cancer-killing features that target cancer cells by inhibiting the key cancer promoting protein, NFkB. Restraining NFkB triggers a process known as apoptosis, which causes the cancer cells to self-destruct.[38-44]

Research has also been done on circulating cancer stem cells (CSCs). These are rogue cells that are not normally detectable or affected by chemo medications. They are responsible for recurrence and relapse in cancer. About 1% of CSCs "travel" in the body. There are currently no drugs to target CSC. In the past five years, delta and gamma have been shown to hinder and control these bad CSCs in cancers of the pancreas, breast, skin, and prostate.[45-50] Amazing that these special forces of vitamin E tocotrienols can do this!

Tocotrienols, especially delta, have shown benefits for recurrent ovarian cancer patients. A study conducted at Denmark's Vejle Hospital and published in *Pharmacological Research* revealed that a combination of delta-tocotrienol and bevacizumab had beneficial effects in chemotherapy for ovarian cancer. This may be due to the anti-angiogenic* activity in delta and bevacizumab. This is the very first clinical trial

---

* Angiogenesis is the growth of new blood vessels. This type of growth is normal and important in fetal development, but it is abnormal in tumors. The new blood vessels that tumors grow steal nutrients from the body to fuel their growth. Anti-angiogenesis is the blocking of new blood vessel growth.

using tocotrienols in ovarian cancer patients that bears a hopeful outcome.

300 mg of tocotrienol were given to advanced stage ovarian cancer patients three times a day along with 10 mg of bevacizumab intravenously every three weeks. The result: 70% disease stabilization (i.e., disease progression was slowed or halted) and an increased survival rate that came very close to doubling.[51]

In 2018, the FDA approved bevacizumab (Avastin®), an anti-angiogenic agent, for treating ovarian cancer after surgery. It was shown to reduce the progression of ovarian cancer by 38% in a double-blind, placebo-controlled study. Results show that with delta-tocotrienol the survival rate for these patients can double (see Figure 5). Truly miraculous!

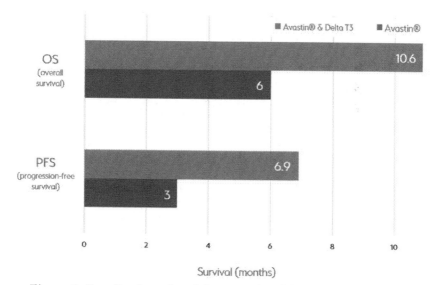

Figure 5: Results show that delta-tocotrienol (in combination with Avastin®) approximately doubled survival rates in patients with recurrent ovarian cancer.

Bone Health (Postmenopausal Osteopenia)

As we age, our bones don't stand much of a chance against free radicals and inflammation. If there was ever a great reason to take antioxidants, it's for our aging bones — including our joints. Many pre-clinical studies have systematically shown promise in this area. [10,11, 52-54]

This is especially helpful for postmenopausal women with osteopenia. Osteopenia is the medical term for the thinning of bone mass, a precursor to the more serious osteoporosis. This is a unique challenge to the "reproductive aging" of menopause where the hormonal makeup changes and a woman's estrogen drops, one of the very few steroid hormones that happens to be an antioxidant. To put it another way — a woman's body reserve of her own endogenous antioxidant is depleted during menopause. If for no other reason, delta-tocotrienol will take the place of estrogen as the "replacement antioxidant."

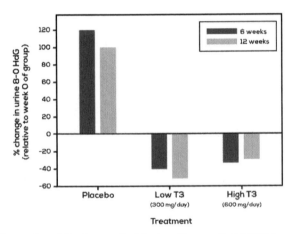

Figure 7: Tocotrienol Reduces Oxidative Stress. 8-OHdG is a breakdown product of DNA, and a biomarker of oxidative stress (oxidative stress has been implicated as one of the contributing factors to bone loss). Tocotrienol reduced oxidative stress, signified by 8-OHdG drop.

A clinical double-blind placebo-controlled trial has been published in regard to this (see Figure 7). Post-menopausal women with osteopenia were given tocopherol-free tocotrienols at two dosages (300 and 600 mg/day) over the course of twelve weeks. This trial showed that tocotrienol decreased bone resorption by 7-24% and improved bone turnover rate by 40-115% simultaneously. This was compared to an independent and blinded control group that was given a placebo. All subjects, including the placebo group, were also given a daily 400 IU vitamin D and 500 mg calcium supplement.[12] So the impact of tocotrienol is above and beyond the known health-related bone properties of vitamin D and calcium.

Delta- and gamma-tocotrienols in many animal studies have already shown promise for strengthening bones, including bones in post-menopausal models with osteopenia.[10,11]

For the record, details of the trial protocol[55] and the safety and FDA approval for the 300 mg/d and 600 mg/d dosages[56] were separately documented.

Alzheimer's Disease (Overall Brain Health)

Cholesterol can play a role in the formation of Alzheimer's disease (AD).[14,57,58] Past studies show tocotrienol – but not tocopherol – to be a promising cholesterol reducer, a feature which may act as an important link to tocotrienol's effect on AD.[5]

Also, tocotrienols, not tocopherols, block the processing of a particular protein associated with helping to "fuel" AD.

In addition, we must not forget the anti-inflammatory activity of tocotrienols, which offers even more protection for brain cells.

Proteins that help brain cells function better require farnesyl pyrophosphate (FPP) and geranylgeranyl pyrophosphate (GGPP). These are "steps" that your body takes to convert simple molecules into something complex that benefits the brain. Tests showed that levels of FPP and GGPP, irrespective of cholesterol levels, were elevated in patients with AD, indicating that they may be directly involved in the disease's progression. When patients took lipid-lowering agents such as statins, however, their risk for cognitive decline was lowered. Tocotrienols may work by decreasing FPP and GGPP, thereby reducing the risk of cognitive decline. Past studies showed various connections between AD reduction and tocotrienols. Tocopherols showed mixed results.[5]

Stroke

When it comes to protecting the brain from further damage from a stroke, researchers at Ohio State University reported in a July 5, 2011 news release that alpha-tocotrienol helps protect brain cells against the aftereffects of a stroke. It does this by increasing the activity of toxin-fighting genes. According to their report, published online in the journal *Stroke*, alpha-tocotrienol can start the production of a protein in the inflamed brain that clears toxins from nerve cells. This prevents cells from dying after a stroke that blocks blood flow.[59] This benefit can be confounded by alpha-tocopherol, the same researchers showed.[60]

In a trial at the Kenneth L. Jordan Research Group in Montclair, New Jersey, researchers discovered tocotrienols' ability to help clear plaque in the carotid artery, thus reducing the risk of stroke. Stroke often occurs when plaque deposits travel upstream and cut off the blood supply to part of the brain.

Fifty individuals with plaque in their arteries were given either 160 mg of gamma- and alpha-tocotrienols a day with 64 mg of alpha-tocopherol in palm oil or a substance with no therapeutic value (placebo). Six months into the study, the dosage in the treatment group was increased to 240 mg of tocotrienols and 96 mg of alpha-tocopherol.

After the research had concluded, ultrasound scans of the carotid artery showed that the plaque had lowered, and the blood flow to the brain had improved in seven of the twenty-five people in the tocotrienol group. The condition had worsened in only two of them. None of the individuals in the placebo group showed any improvement, while ten had gotten worse. No adverse side effects were reported in either group.[61]

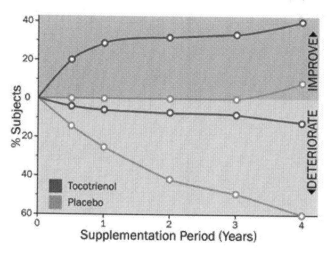

Figure 6

This trial was eventually carried through forty-eight months. Those on 240 mg/day of tocotrienols continued to improve in this time-dependent study. The carotid atherosclerosis in those on placebo progressively got worse (see Figure 6).[62]

Other research studies show vitamin E helps manage high blood pressure, which can result in a stroke.[23,63,64]

NINE

Conditions Tocotrienols Help Manage: Part III

All the Rest

In the beginning of this book, I told you that tocotrienols are not like the typical vitamin E supplement you may have in your home, or that you get from a handful of nuts. In the previous chapters, you have learned a lot about what tocotrienols can do for your health and for disease prevention and/or management. Now let's discover even more benefits of this vitamin.

Arthritis

Arthritis plays no favorites. It doesn't matter if you are strong, weak, young, or old. Did you know that Lucille Ball, Sandy Koufax, and even the famous painter Pierre-Auguste Renoir suffered with rheumatoid arthritis? And that golfer Kristy McPherson and actresses Kathleen Turner and Camryn Manheim still suffer from rheumatoid arthritis today?

An outstanding cause of rheumatoid arthritis and osteoarthritis is inflammation in the unforgiving joints. Delta-tocotrienol may potentially help reduce such inflammation and return mobility.[65]

Eye Health

Delta-tocotrienol may delay the beginning of cataracts when it is applied to the eye. This is likely due to reduced oxidative stress and nitrosative stress to the lenses, which are exposed to environmental oxidants. Nitrosative stress is the reaction of body tissues to nitric acid greater than can be neutralized. These studies were conducted at Universiti Teknologi MARA, Malaysia.[66,67]

In the first study (in rats), researchers tested the effects of annatto tocotrienol on cataract formation, with results showing that tocotrienol slowed cataract onset and progression by reducing oxidative and nitrosative stress. Tocotrienol had a beneficial effect on lens antioxidant enzymes, including superoxide dismutase and catalase, both of which returned to normal levels with the topical treatment. Furthermore, tocotrienol significantly decreased malondialdehyde, a lipid peroxidation end product found to be high in cataracts, and restored the lens soluble to insoluble protein ratio to normal levels.

The study revealed that low doses of tocotrienol in a topical application were most effective, with best outcomes obtained at 0.03% or 300ppm[67].

A second study, using the same eye drop formulation at 0.03% tocotrienol concentration, confirmed that cataract progression was halted with the treatment.[66] In the diabetic rats with advanced-stage cataracts, tocotrienol was able to protect the lens, reducing lens aldose reductase and sorbitol, and reducing inflammation and oxidative stress. Notably, tocotrienol restored lens transparency back to normal, while also improving the lens mitochondrial function.

While previous studies showed that delta-tocotrienol is absorbed in the eye tissue, this is the first study on its beneficial effect on a cataract.[67]

Angiogenesis is the aberrant growth of blood vessels, and is directly involved in eye conditions such as diabetic retinopathy and macular degeneration, which are among the leading causes of blindness. Tocotrienols reduce angiogenesis,[32,68] and hence may slow down angiogenesis-related ocular conditions, including retinopathy and macular degeneration.

Immune System

The immune system is, in a nutshell, a network of white blood cells (WBCs). When you think of your immune system, think of it as a network of "worker ant" WBCs, because if all those cells are not properly protected (from free radicals, toxins, bacteria, viruses, and other invaders getting through the cells' membrane walls), the outcome is uncontrolled invasion.

Like soldiers defending their country, the network works together to defend your body against attacks by invaders. Most of these invaders are microbes — tiny organisms such as bacteria, protozoans, parasites, and fungi that make homes inside your cells and can cause infections. On a good day, when all systems are working, the network removes them.

One study showed that annatto tocotrienol combined with antibiotics had the greatest efficacy in decreasing bacteria when compared with tocotrienol or antibiotic treatment alone. This antimicrobial effect of tocotrienol was strongly associated with increased activity of natural killer cells (a critical part of the immune system) against MRSA, including improved results for repairing wounds.[69]

Taking tocotrienols in this instance would show even stronger beneficial results for the immune system and its T cells. A colleague of mine decided to do a one-person case study with DeltaGold® tocotrienol to assess his T and B lymphocytes in a mitogen-challenge (toxin pathogen secretes). Delta-tocotrienol was the strongest in his "Antioxidant Assay" and the fastest in the "Micronutrient Assay." Interestingly, delta-tocotrienol is complemented by vitamin C as vitamins C & E are known to synergize.[70]

Skin Health

Sun lovers may benefit from antioxidant protection because tocotrienols help reduce damage from ultraviolet rays. And at the same time, these molecules help reduce free radicals created by UV radiation.[71]

In an *in vivo* melanoma study, delta-tocotrienol reduced tumor volume and tumor mass in mice, and significantly delayed tumor progression (significant in that the probability of melanoma development was 3.3-fold higher in the untreated control group). Whereas delta-tocotrienol caused cell death in aberrant melanoma, it did not adversely affect healthy cells.[72]

Even more compelling is the fact that tocotrienol exerts its antitumor activity against melanoma by targeting cancer stem cells.[50]

In other studies conducted at the University of Wisconsin/Madison and at the Texas Woman's University, cell cultures and animal studies showed that gamma- and delta-tocotrienols helped stop the growth of melanoma.[43,73,74]

Vitamin E has long been lauded for its skin health benefits. Although quantitatively, alpha-tocopherol comprises the bulk of vitamin E found in the epidermis, tocotrienols — applied orally or topically — also deliver to viable skin layers.[75,76] In this context, tocotrienols have been found to reduce hyperpigmentation,[77] repair skin damage, heal wounds,[78] protect from light exposure,[79] and suppress skin cancer.[73]

Of the various E vitamers, delta- and gamma-tocotrienols were the most potent in reducing skin pigmentation and blemishes by inhibiting melanin synthesis.[79] Delta-tocotrienol was also shown to suppress melanoma.[73] The SPF value of delta-tocotrienol was reported to be 5.5.[79]

Radiation Poisoning

If I add to all I have said already and tell you that tocotrienols have been shown to help guard against radiation, it might seem as if I am making these molecules out to be too good to be true. I must say that I was in disbelief myself. But, even the Armed Forces Radiobiology Research Institute (AFRRI) of the Uniformed Services University (Bethesda, MD) looked at tocotrienols as a radiation countermeasure agent.[80]

Of the hundreds of agents studied, gamma- and delta-tocotrienol remained as radiation countermeasure agents of interest.

AFRRI conducted this research on tocotrienols because these molecules were found to be the most effective natural form of radioprotectors. But only delta and gamma work effectively.[81,82] When animals were subjected to whole-body radiation (with intention to kill), both tocotrienols extended survival unambiguously.

AFRRI has roughly twenty published studies on tocotrienols and radiation protection, including GI tract protection, and remobilization of blood cells. It is remarkable to see that delta and gamma are able to salvage healthy cells from severe ionization radiation[†].

The research is intended to discover ways to protect our armed forces when they are placed in harm's way.

I believe these studies have another useful, civilian purpose. Delta-tocotrienol and gamma-tocotrienol may help patients who are undergoing oncologic radiotherapy.

[†] Ionizing radiation means destructive radiation that induces massive reactive oxygen species, a tsunami of inflammation, and often certain death. This is so destructive it is often irreversible. At best, we can only minimize and mitigate damage.

TEN

Protocol: How to Get the Best Results from Tocotrienol

By now I hope you have a better understanding of the many benefits of annatto tocotrienols. But, of course, you undoubtedly have questions. Here are some common questions and answers.

How much should a normal healthy person take?

100-200 mg of tocotrienol per day is adequate for lipid antioxidant protection for all cell membranes and lipoproteins.

The annatto tocotrienol known as DeltaGold® was granted FDA-affirmed GRAS in 2014 and has been proven safe in a variety of clinical trials up to 600 mg/day.

Studies estimate the safe dose of tocotrienols for humans may be as high as 1,000 mg/day.

Can I get enough tocotrienol from my diet?

Unfortunately, no. The average American diet only provides 2 mg of tocotrienol per day, a mere 1-2% of the expected daily amount. Therefore, supplementation is needed to obtain adequate antioxidant protection.

How much should a condition-specific person take?

The recommended dose for a person with a mild chronic condition is 300-450 mg per day, and for a person with an advanced chronic condition, 450-600 mg per day. Clinical trials indicate that the highest dose taken safely for 24 months is 900 mg per day. Most indications call for 300-600 mg per day dosages.

When should I take tocotrienol?

Tocotrienol is lipid soluble so it is best consumed with a meal. Up to 300 mg of tocotrienol can be taken at each meal to allow the ease of absorption. Higher doses should be taken apart at different meals. It should not be taken on an empty stomach.

Do I need to worry about dietary alpha-tocopherol?

If you are referring to the interference that alpha-tocopherol would have on tocotrienols, then tocopherols coming from a healthy diet will not show any interference to tocotrienols. It is only when tocopherols are 15% of total vitamin E amount that they start to interfere with the functions of the tocotrienols.

If you are concerned about getting enough alpha-tocopherol in your diet, adding a few ounces of nuts or sunflower seeds, and/or a few tablespoons of vegetable oil such as wheat germ oil, sunflower, or safflower, to your healthy diet should suffice.

Will supplementing alpha-tocopherol interfere?

Yes, supplementing alpha-tocopherol will interfere with tocotrienol benefits. But don't worry, there is usually no need to supplement alpha-tocopherol as you likely obtain the recommended 15 mg/day through diet alone.

Can I take DeltaGold® while on my prescriptions?

There is usually no contraindication to tocotrienol usage with medicines, although it is wise to consult with your healthcare professional before starting any nutritional supplement plan.

Because tocotrienols have up to fifty times the antioxidant potential that tocopherols have, do I still need to eat antioxidant foods?

Tocotrienols are not meant to replace antioxidant foods. Tocotrienols enhance your diet for better health. Supplements are called "supplements" for a reason, they are not called "substitutions." You should always try to eat a variety of healthy, whole foods.

Is DeltaGold® really that effective as an antioxidant?

In studies at Brunswick Laboratories, Dr. Boxin Ou compared the ORAC value of DeltaGold® to tocopherol and mixed tocotrienols, and found that the antioxidant potential from DeltaGold® is much higher than that of the other compounds studied.

In addition, Ohio State University found that delta- and gamma-tocotrienol (as in DeltaGold®) protect lard from oxidation at low levels of just 100 ppm. The USDA lab and University of Georgia both published articles stating that DeltaGold® is effective in protecting fats in deep frying and omega-3s in infant formulas.[83,84]

Dr. Lester Packer of the University of California/Berkeley also showed that, as antioxidants, tocotrienols are 40-60 times more potent than tocopherols.[4]

In clinical studies delta-tocotrienol increased other endogenous antioxidants.[85]

Should tocotrienol softgels be refrigerated?

Tocotrienols are very stable and tocotrienol in softgels are even more stable. They remain at the same potency for at least three years at room temperature. Refrigeration is not necessary.

What other supplements can I take with DeltaGold®?

You want to think about antioxidants and anti-inflammatories — in addition to compounds for your immune and cardio system. A diet of fish, kale, carrots, oatmeal, other nutritious cereals, citrus fruits, and dairy can give you almost what you need. But here's a starter list to go by if you are looking for supplements:

Conditions	Daily Tocotrienol Recommended Dosage*	Supplement Complement Toco...
Inflammation	250 mg	CoQ10, Omega-3 fatty acids, Alpha-lipoic acid, Curcumin, Resveratrol
High lipids	250 mg	Niacin, Omega-3 fatty acids, Psyllium, Red yeast rice
Arthritis	250 mg	CoQ10, Omega-3 fatty acids, Glucosamine, Chondroitin
Cancer	400-900 mg	Vitamins C, D, Selenium, B complex
Cardiovascular disease & MetS	250 mg	CoQ10, Omega-3 fatty acids, Magnesium, Resveratrol, Red yeast rice, MK4, MK7
Eye health	N/A	Lutein, Zeaxanthin, Omega-3 fatty acids, Vitamins A, C, Zinc
Immune system	N/A	Zinc, Vitamins B6, B12, C, D
Bone health	300 mg	Vitamins D, Calcium, MK4
Alzheimer's Brain health	~350 mg	Omega-3 fatty acids, Vitamins B12 and C, Resveratrol, Alpha-GPC**
Asthma	N/A	Vitamin D
Skin health	N/A	Vitamins A, C, Zinc, Selenium
Radiation damage	400-600 mg	Iodine, Genistein
NAFLD "Fatty Liver"	600 mg	CoQ10, Omega-3, Methionine, Glutathione

*Up to 300 mg of tocotrienol can be taken at each meal. Higher doses should be taken apart at different meals.
**L-alpha glycerylphosphorylcholine (Alpha-GPC)
For more FAQs: http://americanrivernutrition.com/faqs

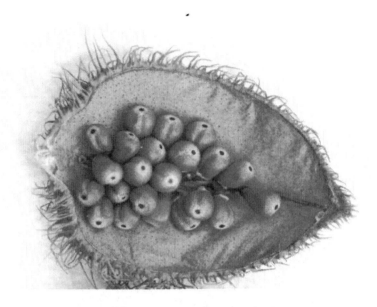

Learn More • BarrieTan.com

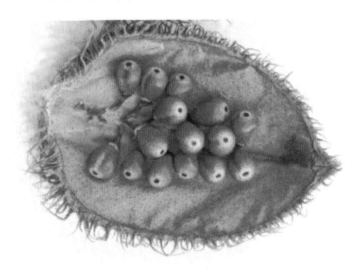

References:

1. Eva Bianconi, Allison Piovesan, Federica Facchin, Alina Beraudi, Raffaella Casadei, Flavia Frabetti, Lorenza Vitale, Maria Chiara Pelleri, Simone Tassani, Francesco Piva, Soledad Perez-Amodio, Pierluigi Strippoli & Silvia Canaider (2013) "An estimation of the number of cells in the human body." *Annals of Human Biology*, 40:6, 463-471, DOI: 10.3109/03014460.2013.807878

2. Madrigal, Alexis (2009, September 9). "Humans have made, found or used over 50 million unique chemicals." Retrieved from https://www.wired.com/2009/09/humans-have-made-found-or-used-over-50-million-unique-chemicals/

3. Olcott, H. S. & Emerson, O. H. (1937). "Antioxidants and the autoxidation of fats." IX. "The antioxidant properties of the tocopherols." *Journal of the American Chemical Society*,59:1008–1009.

4. Serbinova E, Kagan V, Han D, Packer L. "Free radical recycling and intramembrane mobility in the antioxidant properties of alpha-tocopherol and alpha-tocotrienol." *Free Radical Biology & Medicine*, 1991;10(5):263-75.

5. Xia W, Mo H. "Potential of tocotrienols in the prevention and therapy of Alzheimer's disease." *Journal of Nutritional Biochemistry*, 2016;31:1-9. Epub 2016/05/03.

6. Mangialasche F, Kivipelto M, Mecocci P, Rizzuto D, Palmer K, Winblad B, et al. "High plasma levels of vitamin E forms and reduced Alzheimer's disease risk in advanced age." *Journal of Alzheimer's Disease,* JAD. 2010;20(4):1029-37. Epub 2010/04/24.

7. Mangialasche F, Xu W, Kivipelto M, Costanzi E, Ercolani S, Pigliautile M, et al. "Tocopherols and tocotrienols plasma levels are associated with cognitive impairment." *Neurobiology of Aging,* 2012;33(10):2282-90. Epub 2011/12/24.

8. Mangialasche F, Westman E, Kivipelto M, Muehlboeck JS, Cecchetti R, Baglioni M, et al. "Classification and prediction of clinical diagnosis of Alzheimer's disease based on MRI and plasma measures of alpha-/gamma-tocotrienols and gamma-tocopherol." *Journal of Internal Medicine,* 2013. Epub 2013/01/25.

9. Mangialasche F, Solomon A, Kareholt I, Hooshmand B, Cecchetti R, Fratiglioni L, et al. "Serum levels of vitamin E forms and risk of cognitive impairment in a Finnish cohort of older adults." *Experimental Gerontology,* 2013;48(12):1428-35. Epub 2013/10/12.

10. Chin, K.Y., et al. "The Effects of Tocotrienol and Lovastatin Co-Supplementation on Bone Dynamic Histomorphometry and Bone Morphogenetic Protein-2 Expression in Rats with Estrogen Deficiency." *Nutrients,* 2017. 9(2).

11. Chin, K.Y., et al. "The Effects of Annatto Tocotrienol on Bone Biomechanical Strength and Bone Calcium Content

in an Animal Model of Osteoporosis Due to Testosterone Deficiency." *Nutrients*, 2016. 8(12).

12. Shen, C.L., et al. "Tocotrienol supplementation suppressed bone resorption and oxidative stress in postmenopausal osteopenic women: a 12-week randomized double-blinded placebo-controlled trial." *Osteoporos International*, 2018.

13. Qureshi, A.A., et al. "Impact of delta-tocotrienol on inflammatory biomarkers and oxidative stress in hypercholesterolemic subjects." *Journal of Clinical & Experimental Cardiology*, 2015. 6(4): p. 1000367.

14. Qureshi AA, Khan DA, Mahjabeen W, Qureshi N. "Dose-dependent modulation of lipid parameters, cytokines, and RNA by delta-tocotrienol in hypercholesterolemic subjects restricted to AHA Step-1 diet." *British Journal of Medicine and Medical Research*, 2015;6(4):351-66.

15. Qureshi AA, Khan DA, Mahjabeen W, Papasian CJ, Qureshi N. "Nutritional supplement-5 with a combination of proteasome inhibitors (resveratrol, quercetin, delta-tocotrienol) modulate age-associated biomarkers and cardiovascular lipid parameters in human subjects." *Journal of Clinical & Experimental Cardiology*. 2013;4(3):1-14.

16. Qureshi AA, Khan DA, Mahjabeen W, Papasian CJ, Qureshi N (2012) "Suppression of nitric oxide production and cardiovascular risk factors in healthy seniors and hypercholesterolemic subjects by a combination of polyphenols and vitamins." *Journal of Clinical & Experimental Cardiology*, S5:008. doi:10.4172/2155-9880.S5-008

17. Pearce BC, Parker RA, Deason ME, Qureshi AA, Wright JJ. "Hypocholesterolemic activity of synthetic and natural tocotrienols." *Journal of Medicinal Chemistry*, 1992;35:3595-606.

18. Parker RA, Pearce BC, Clark RW, Gordon DA, Wright JJ. "Tocotrienols regulate cholesterol production in mammalian cells by post-transcriptional suppression of 3-hydroxy-3-methylglutaryl-coenzyme A reductase." *Journal of Biological Chemistry*, 1993;268:11230-8.

19. Song BL, DeBose-Boyd RA. "Insig-dependent ubiquitination and degradation of 3-hydroxy-3-methylglutaryl coenzyme a reductase stimulated by delta- and gamma-tocotrienols." *Journal of Biological Chemistry*, 2006. 281:25054-61.

20. Zaiden N, Yap WN, Ong S, Xu CH, Teo VH, Chang CP, et al. "Gamma delta tocotrienols reduce hepatic triglyceride synthesis and VLDL secretion." *Journal of Atherosclerosis and Thrombosis*. 2010;17(10):1019-32.

21. O'Byrne D, Grundy S, Packer L, Devaraj S, Baldenius K, Hoppe PP, et al. Studies of LDL oxidation following alpha-, gamma-, or delta-tocotrienyl acetate supplementation of hypercholesterolemic humans. *Free Radical Biology & Medicine*, 2000;29(9):834-45.

22. Carr AC, Zhu BZ, Frei B. "Potential antiatherogenic mechanisms of ascorbate (vitamin C) and alpha-tocopherol (vitamin E)." Circ Res. 2000;87(5):349-54. Epub 2000/09/02.

23. Wong, W.Y., et al. "Anti-inflammatory gamma- and delta-tocotrienols improve cardiovascular, liver and metabolic

function in diet-induced obese rats." *European Journal of Nutrition,* 2017. 56(1): p. 133-150.

24. Allen L, Ramalingam L, Menikdiwela K, Scoggin S, Shen CL, Tomison MD, et al. "Effects of delta-tocotrienol on obesity-related adipocyte hypertrophy, inflammation and hepatic steatosis in high-fat-fed mice." *Journal of Nutritional Biochemistry,* 2017;48:128-37. Epub 2017/08/22.

25. Buckner T, Fan R, Kim Y, Kim J, Chung S. Annatto Tocotrienol Attenuates NLRP3 "Inflammasome Activation in Macrophages." *Current Developments in Nutrition,* 2017;1(6):e000760. Epub 2018/06/30.

26. Shibata A, Kawakami Y, Kimura T, Miyazawa T, Nakagawa K. "Alpha-Tocopherol Attenuates the Triglyceride- and Cholesterol-Lowering Effects of Rice Bran Tocotrienol in Rats Fed a Western Diet." *Journal of Agricultural and Food Chemistry,* 2016;64(26):5361-6. Epub 2016/06/14.

27. Le, M., Devaki, P., Ha, N., Jun, D., Te, H., Cheung, R. and Nguyen, M. (2017). *Prevalence of non-alcoholic fatty liver disease and risk factors for advanced fibrosis and mortality in the United States.* PLOS. Available from: https://journals.plos.org/plosone/article?id=10.1371/journal.pone.0173499.

28. Estes, C., Razavi, H., Loomba, R., Younossi, Z. and Sanyal, A. (2018). "Modeling the Epidemic of Nonalcoholic Fatty Liver Disease Demonstrates an Exponential Increase in Burden of Disease." *Hepatology,* 67(1).

29. Pervez, M.A., et al. "Effects of Delta-tocotrienol Supplementation on Liver Enzymes, Inflammation, Oxidative stress and Hepatic Steatosis in Patients with Nonalcoholic Fatty Liver Disease." *Turkish Journal of Gastroenterology*, 2018. 29(2): p. 170-176.

30. Fang F, Kang Z, Wong C. "Vitamin E tocotrienols improve insulin sensitivity through activating peroxisome proliferator-activated receptors." *Molecular Nutrition and Food Research*, October, 2009 at Guangzhou Institute of Biomedicine and Health, Chinese Academy of Sciences, Guangzhou Science City, Guangzhou, P. R. China.

31. Elson, C.E. "Suppression of mevalonate pathway activities by dietary isoprenoids: protective roles in cancer and cardiovascular disease." *Journal of Nutrition*, 1995. 125(6 Suppl): p. 1666S-1672S.

32. Miyazawa, T., et al. "Anti-angiogenic function of tocotrienol." *Asia Pacific Journal of Clinical Nutrition*, 2008. 17 Suppl 1: p. 253-6.

33. Nakagawa, K., et al. "DNA chip analysis of comprehensive food function: inhibition of angiogenesis and telomerase activity with unsaturated vitamin E, tocotrienol." *Biofactors*, 2004. 21(1-4): p. 5-10.

34. McIntyre BS, Briski KP, Gapor A, Sylvester PW. "Antiproliferative and apoptotic effects of tocopherols and tocotrienols on preneoplastic and neoplastic mouse mammary epithelial cells." *Proceedings of the Society of Experimental Biology and Medicine*, 2000;224(4):292-301.

35. Khallouki F, de Medina P, Caze-Subra S, Bystricky K, Balaguer P, Poirot M, et al. "Molecular and Biochemical Analysis of the Estrogenic and Proliferative Properties of Vitamin E Compounds." *Frontiers in Oncology,* 2015;5:287. Epub 2016/01/19.

36. Mo H, Elson CE. "Studies of the isoprenoid-mediated inhibition of mevalonate synthesis applied to cancer chemotherapy and chemoprevention." *Experimental Biology and Medicine,* 2004(229):567-85.

37. Hindler K, Cleeland CS, Rivera E, Collard CD. "The role of statins in cancer therapy." *The Oncologist,* 2006;11(3):306-15. Epub 2006/03/22.

38. Montagnani Marelli M, Marzagalli M, Moretti RM, Beretta G, Casati L, Comitato R, et al. "Vitamin E delta-tocotrienol triggers endoplasmic reticulum stress-mediated apoptosis in human melanoma cells." *Scientific Reports,* 2016;6:30502. Epub 2016/07/28.

39. Jiang Q. "Natural forms of vitamin E and metabolites-regulation of cancer cell death and underlying mechanisms." IUBMB Life. 2019;71(4):495-506. Epub 2018/12/15.

40. Yang C, Jiang Q. "Vitamin E delta-tocotrienol inhibits TNF-alpha-stimulated NF-kappaB activation by up-regulation of anti-inflammatory A20 via modulation of sphingolipid including elevation of intracellular dihydroceramides." *Journal of Nutritional Biochemistry,* 2019;64:101-9. Epub 2018/11/25.

41. Qureshi AA, Zuvanich EG, Khan DA, Mushtaq S, Silswal N, Qureshi N. "Proteasome inhibitors modulate anticancer and anti-proliferative properties via NF-kB signaling, and ubiquitin-proteasome pathways in cancer cell lines of different organs." *Lipids in Health and Disease*, 2018;17(1):62. Epub 2018/04/03.

42. Nesaretnam K, Meganathan P. "Tocotrienols: inflammation and cancer." *Annals of the New York Academy of Scientists*, 2011;1229(1):18-22.

43. He L, Mo H, Hadisusilo S, Qureshi AA, Elson CE. "Isoprenoids suppress the growth of murine B16 melanomas in vitro and in vivo." *Journal of Nutrition*, 1997;127(5):668-74.

44. Fernandes NV, Guntipalli PK, Mo H. "d-delta-Tocotrienol-mediated cell cycle arrest and apoptosis in human melanoma cells." *Anticancer Research,* 2010;30(12):4937-44. Epub 2010/12/29.

45. Luk SU, Yap WN, Chiu YT, Lee DT, Ma S, Lee TK, et al. "Gamma-tocotrienol as an effective agent in targeting prostate cancer stem cell-like population." *Int J Cancer.* 2011;128(9):2182-91.

46. Kaneko S, Sato C, Shiozawa N, Sato A, Sato H, Virgona N, et al. "Suppressive Effect of Delta-Tocotrienol on Hypoxia Adaptation of Prostate Cancer Stem-like Cells." *Anticancer research.* 2018;38(3):1391-9. Epub 2018/03/02.

47. Gopalan A, Yu W, Sanders BG, Kline K. "Eliminating drug resistant breast cancer stem-like cells with combination of

simvastatin and gamma-tocotrienol." *Cancer Lett.* 2013;328(2):285-96. Epub 2012/10/16.

48. Xiong A, Yu W, Tiwary R, Sanders BG, Kline K. "Distinct roles of different forms of vitamin E in DHA-induced apoptosis in triple-negative breast cancer cells." *Mol Nutr Food Res.* 2012;56(6):923-34. Epub 2012/06/19.

49. Husain K, Centeno BA, Coppola D, Trevino J, Sebti SM, Malafa MP. "delta-Tocotrienol, a natural form of vitamin E, inhibits pancreatic cancer stem-like cells and prevents pancreatic cancer metastasis." *Oncotarget.* 2017;8(19):31554-67. Epub 2017/04/14.

50. Marzagalli M, Moretti RM, Messi E, Marelli MM, Fontana F, Anastasia A, et al. "Targeting melanoma stem cells with the Vitamin E derivative delta-tocotrienol." *Scientific reports.* 2018;8(1):587. Epub 2018/01/14.

51. Thomsen CB, Andersen RF, Steffensen KD, Adimi P, Jakobsen, A. "Delta tocotrienol in recurrent ovarian cancer. A phase II trial." *Pharmacological Research,* 2019;141:392-6. Epub 2019/01/15.

52. Chin, K.Y. and S. Ima-Nirwana, "Effects of annatto-derived tocotrienol supplementation on osteoporosis induced by testosterone deficiency in rats." *Clinical Interventions in Aging,* 2014. 9: p. 1247-59.

53. Chin, K.Y. and S. Ima-Nirwana, "The biological effects of tocotrienol on bone: a review on evidence from rodent models." *Drug Design, Development and Therapy,* 2015. 9: p. 2049-61.

54. Shen, C.L., et al. "Tocotrienols for bone health: a translational approach." *Annals of the New York Academy of Scientists,* 2017. 1401(1): p. 150-165.

55. Shen CL, Mo H, Yang S, Wang S, Felton CK, Tomison MD, et al. "Safety and efficacy of tocotrienol supplementation for bone health in postmenopausal women: protocol for a dose-response double-blinded placebo-controlled randomised trial." *BMJ Open.* 2016;6(12):e012572. Epub 2016/12/25.

56. Shen CL, Wang S, Yang S, Tomison MD, Abbasi M, Hao L, et al. "A 12-week evaluation of annatto tocotrienol supplementation for postmenopausal women: safety, quality of life, body composition, physical activity, and nutrient intake." *BMC Complementary and Alternative Medicine,* 2018;18(1):198. Epub 2018/06/30.

57. Yu SG, Thomas AM, Gapor A, Tan B, Qureshi N, Qureshi AA. "Dose-response impact of various tocotrienols on serum lipid parameters in 5-week-old female chickens." *Lipids.* 2006;41(5):453-61.

58. Y. Qureshi AA, Pearce BC, Nor RM, Gapor A, Peterson DM, Elson CE. "Dietary alpha-tocopherol attenuates the impact of gamma-tocotrienol on hepatic 3-hydroxy-3-methylglutaryl coenzyme A reductase activity in chickens." *J Nutr.* 1996;126(2):389-94.

59. Rink C, Christoforidis G, Khanna S, Peterson L, Patel Y, Abduljalil A, et al. "Tocotrienol vitamin E protects against preclinical canine ischemic stroke by inducing arteriogenesis. Journal of cerebral blood flow and

metabolism." *Official Journal of the International Society of Cerebral Blood Flow and Metabolism,* 2011;31(11):2218-30. Epub 2011/06/16.

60. Khanna S, Heigel M, Weist J, Gnyawali S, Teplitsky S, Roy S, et al. "Excessive alpha-tocopherol exacerbates microglial activation and brain injury caused by acute ischemic stroke." *Faseb* J. 2014. Epub 2014/11/21.

61. Tomeo AC, Geller M, Watkins TR, Gapor A, Bierenbaum ML. "Antioxidant effects of tocotrienols in patients with hyperlipidemia and carotid stenosis." *Lipids,* 1995 Dec;30(12):1179-83.

62. Kooyenga DK, Watson TR, Geller M, Bierenbaum M. "Antioxidants modulate the course of carotid atherosclerosis: A four-year report." In: Nesaretnam K, Packer L, editors. *Micronutrients and Health,* Illinois: AOCS Press; 2001. p. 366-75.

63. Newaz MA, Nawal NN. "Effect of gamma-tocotrienol on blood pressure, lipid peroxidation and total antioxidant status in spontaneously hypertensive rats (SHR)." *Clinical and Experimental Hypertension,* 1999;21(8):1297-313.

64. Newaz MA, Yousefipour Z, Nawal N, Adeeb N. "Nitric oxide synthase activity in blood vessels of spontaneously hypertensive rats: antioxidant protection by gamma-tocotrienol." *Journal of Physiology and Pharmacology,* 2003;54(3):319-27.

65. Haleagrahara N, Swaminathan M, Chakravarthi S, Radhakrishnan A. "Therapeutic Efficacy of Vitamin E delta-Tocotrienol in Collagen-Induced Rat Model of

Arthritis." *BioMed Research International,* 2014;2014:539540. Epub 2014/08/13.

66. Abdul Nasir NA, Agarwal R, Sheikh Abdul Kadir SH, Vasudevan S, Tripathy M, Iezhitsa I, et al. "Reduction of oxidative-nitrosative stress underlies anticataract effect of topically applied tocotrienol in streptozotocin-induced diabetic rats." *PLOS One,* 2017;12(3):e0174542. Epub 2017/03/30.

67. Abdul Nasir NA, Agarwal R, Vasudevan S, Tripathy M, Alyautdin R, Ismail NM. "Effects of Topically Applied Tocotrienol on Cataractogenesis and Lens Redox Status in galactosemic rats." *Molecular Vision,* 2014 Jun 12;20:822-35. eCollection 2014.

68. Shibata, A., et al. "Tumor anti-angiogenic effect and mechanism of action of delta-tocotrienol." *Biochemical Pharmacology,* 2008. 76(3): p. 330-9.

69. Pierpaoli E, Orlando F, Cirioni O, Simonetti O, Giacometti A, Provinciali M. "Supplementation with tocotrienols from Bixa orellana improves the in vivo efficacy of daptomycin against methicillin-resistant Staphylococcus aureus in a mouse model of infected wound." *Phytomedicine,* 2017;36:50-3. Epub 2017/11/22.

70. Kagan VE, Serbinova EA, Forte T, Scita G, Packer L. "Recycling of vitamin E in human low density lipoproteins." Journal of Lipid Research, 1992;33(3):385-97. Epub 1992/03/01.

71. Kagan V, Witt E, Goldman R, Scita G, Packer L. "Ultraviolet light-induced generation of vitamin E radicals

and their recycling. A possible photosensitizing effect of vitamin E in skin." *Free Radical Research Communications*, 1992;16(1):51-64. Epub 1992/01/01.

72. Montagnani Marelli M, Marzagalli M, Moretti RM, Beretta G, Casati L, Comitato R, et al. "Vitamin E delta-tocotrienol triggers endoplasmic reticulum stress-mediated apoptosis in human melanoma cells." *Scientific Reports,* 2016;6:30502. Epub 2016/07/28.

73. Fernandes NV, Guntipalli PK, Mo H. "d-delta-Tocotrienol-mediated cell cycle arrest and apoptosis in human melanoma cells." *Anticancer Research*, 30(12):4937-44.

74. McAnally JA, Gupta J, Sodhani S, Bravo L, Mo H. "Tocotrienols potentiate lovastatin-mediated growth suppression in vitro and in vivo." *Experimental Biology and Medicine (Maywood),* 2007 Apr;232(4):523-31.

75. Fuchs J, Weber S, Podda M, Groth N, Herrling T, Packer L, et al. "HPLC analysis of vitamin E isoforms in human epidermis: correlation with minimal erythema dose and free radical scavenging activity." *Free Radical Biological Medicine,* 2003;34(3):330-6. Epub 2003/01/25.

76. Traber, M. G., M. Podda, et al. (1997). "Diet-derived and topically applied tocotrienols accumulate in skin and protect the tissue against ultraviolet light-induced oxidative stress." *Asia Pacific Journal of Clinical Nutrition*, 6(1): 63-67.

77. Michihara, A., Morita, S., Hirokawa, Y., Ago, K., & Tsuji, H. (2009). "Delta-tocotrienol causes decrease of melanin

content in mouse melanoma cells." *Journal of Health Sciences*, 55(2), 314-318.

78. Musalmah M, Nizrana MY, Fairuz AH, NoorAini AH, Azian AL, Gapor MT, et al. "Comparative effects of palm vitamin E and alpha-tocopherol on healing and wound tissue antioxidant enzyme levels in diabetic rats." *Lipids*, 2005;40(6):575-80. Epub 2005/09/10.

79. Yap, W. N., N. Zaiden, et al. (2010). "Gamma- and delta-tocotrienols inhibit skin melanin synthesis by suppressing constitutive and UV-induced tyrosinase activation." *Pigment Cell & Melanoma Research*, 23(5): 688-692.

80. Institute, A.F.R.R. *Radiation Countermeasures*. 2011 6/14/2011; Available from: http://www.usuhs.mil/afrri/research/rcp.htm.

81. Kulkarni, S., et al. "Gamma-tocotrienol protects hematopoietic stem and progenitor cells in mice after total-body irradiation." *Radiat Research*, 2010. 173(6): p. 738-47.

82. Li, X.H., et al. "Delta-tocotrienol protects mouse and human hematopoietic progenitors from gamma-irradiation through extracellular signal-regulated kinase/mammalian target of rapamycin signaling." *Haematologica*, 95(12): p. 1996-2004.

83. Winkler-Moser JK, Bakota EL, Hwang HS. "Stability and Antioxidant Activity of Annatto (Bixa orellana L.) Tocotrienols During Frying and in Fried Tortilla Chips." *J Food Science and Technology*, 2018;83(2):266-74. Epub 2018/01/18.

84. Zou L, Akoh CC. "Antioxidant activities of annatto and palm tocotrienol-rich fractions in fish oil and structured lipid-based infant formula emulsion." *Food Chemistry*, 2015;168:504-11. Epub 2014/08/31.

85. Tan B, Mueller AM. "Tocotrienols in Cardiometabolic Diseases." In: Watson R, Preedy V, editors. *Tocotrienols: Vitamin E beyond Tocopherol*: AOCS/CRC Press; 2008. p. 257-73.

53524364R00052

Made in the
USA
Lexington, KY